MW01195623

Back to the Basics

Life Revitalization through Bio-Identical Hormones

Greg Brannon, M.D.

Greg Brannon, M.D. and *The Youth Institute*

Table of Contents

Dedication

First and foremost,

To my best friend and the biggest supporter of my life,

my wife, Jody.

I also want to dedicate this book to future knowledge seekers.

*Remember: **Knowledge is power!***

Don't be afraid to question everything.

May this book cause you to study deeper,

research more thoroughly, and push harder for the truth.

Liberty always requires responsibility.

Forward by Charles Rizzuto, M.D.

As an anesthesiologist, I am an expert in human physiology and the pharmaceuticals .that are available to modern medicine. I safely navigate patients through complex procedures keeping their bodies in perfect homeostasis for the duration of the surgery.

I care for patients with a wide range of medical conditions. Their health affected by their lifestyle, genetics, environmental exposures and the process of aging. Dr. Greg Brannon maintains that many of the common changes we see as one ages are not normal. These changes are mostly attributed to decreasing levels of hormones.

Dr. Brannon, a dear friend of mine for over thirty years, clearly explains these changes that occur in both men and women. As an OB-GYN for over twenty-five years, he is an expert in the hormonal changes that occur in one's lifetime. Dr. Brannon graduated from the University of Southern California in 1982. He graduated from The University of Health and Science Chicago Medical School in 1988 and completed his residency in OB-GYN at the University of Southern California Women's Hospital in 1992. He has taught as a clinical associate professor at the University of North Carolina School of Medicine and has been in private practice in the Raleigh-Durham area since 1993. Dr. Brannon lives in North Carolina with his lovely wife Jody, where they have raised seven children.

In the following pages, Dr. Brannon explores the common changes we see with aging. He emphasizes that *"common is not normal."* He describes how hormones work. As we age, the levels of important hormones decrease. He explains the various causes of these decreases. He describes what happens to the body as we correct these deficiencies with bio-identical hormone replacement therapy (BHRT). He explains how synthetic hormone replacement differs from BHRT. He acknowledges the controversies surrounding replacement therapy but cites multiple research articles to support his practice. He speaks about the advantages of pellet replacement therapy over other forms. He explains how the procedure is performed and why it is the preferred method of medication administration for a smoother onset and longer steady state of blood level concentrations. His many success stories of patients whose lives have been greatly impacted illustrate how Dr. Brannon puts his talent and great knowledge to work.

Dr. Brannon is the Medical Director at *The Youth Institute* in Cary, North Carolina. He concludes by explaining how one can get started with bio-identical hormone replacement by an expert in the field.

Introduction

Knowledge is power.

When you have knowledge about how your body works and how to get your life back, you have *power*.

How much do you know about how your body functions? How in-tune are you with what's going on inside of you? Do you know the basic principles of hormones and how they relate to your health?

You are about to discover some of the best research available about how to maintain maximum health and vitality as you age – through Bio-identical Hormone Replacement Therapy (BHRT).

BHRT is not new. As you can see from the cover of this book, it's been around a long time … since the 1930s. Those early researchers and proponents knew something very profound: *often you have to go back to the basics to get something right.*

The goal of this book is to go back to the basics of health optimization and help you get your life back!

A wise man once said, *"We do not become conscious of the three greatest blessings of life, such as health, youth, and freedom, as long as we possess them, but only after we have lost them."* [i]

One thing many people have lost today is the blessing of good health. Our bodies have changed. Whether you are facing depression, low energy, poor focus, low libido, or a myriad of other diseases and symptoms, people are not aging gracefully anymore. And it's not just those in their forties and older. I'm seeing many younger men and women with hormone deficiencies that take their toll on those in their twenties.

Throughout this book, I want you to look at the over-whelming amount of research that will show the positive effects of *Bio-identical Hormone Replacement Therapy*. When our hormone levels return to normal levels – to where they *should be* – our bodies will be strengthened and have the best chance to age gracefully and stay healthy and strong.

Everything I teach is backed-up by medical research, white papers, and scientific studies. I will mention some of this research throughout this book – but because it is, by nature, an introduction, I will also point you to extensive amounts of research that is available on our web site.

I also understand there is a degree of controversy over hormone replacement therapy. There are experts on each side. And it is up to you, the individual, to do your own research and come to your own conclusions about what is best for you.

My Personal Motivation

In this book, I am speaking for myself. My convictions come from years of study, reading research papers, and years of clinical practice.

Those who know me well know that I have always followed a path of questioning everything. I've asked questions like, *"Why are we sick?"* *"Why are there chronic diseases?"* *"Why are there complications today that we have not seen in the past?"*

I want to look for the *cause*, not just the *cure*. In finding the right cause for what ails us, we may find the best cure. I'm looking for remedies that will help the individual. And I am on a quest to help each individual according to their health-related needs and their wants. I believe the individual is the final authority over their health care.

The Case for Bio-identical Hormones

Come join me in this journey and let me convince you why bio-identical hormone treatment is for you. Let me take you back to the basics of hormonal balance, drawing on thousands of research papers and studies to show that bio-identical hormones are safe, proven, and effective.

So why is there so much controversy surrounding hormones?

It is important to understand the *Center for Disease Control* (CDC) and the *Federal Drug Administration* (FDA) group all types of hormones together. In their mind, there is no difference between synthetic and bio-identical hormones. They group them together in the same category ... and therefore, what is dangerous for one type of hormone is, by association, true of the other.

Seriously? People actually make that false assumption?

I disagree with those organizations ... wholeheartedly!

Let me give you just one example why. These governmental regulatory agencies call both "natural progesterone" and "medroxyprogesterone" (MPA) *"progestins."* But these two progestins are very different. They may act somewhat alike, but there is a world of difference in terms of their chemical make-up, how they are produced, where they come from, and how the body responds to them.

How important is this? It's a matter of life-and-death! Studies have shown that the natural progesterone may actually *decrease* the likelihood of breast cancer, while another progestin, synthetic MPA, may actually *increase* its likelihood by up to 69%.

Just because a hormone is labeled a progestin doesn't make it safe. Neither does it necessarily make it dangerous. We must look at the source and structure of that hormone.

- If the source is foreign to the human body, we must ask if it presents dangers and harmful repercussions.
- If the source is your own body, it makes sense that the body would receive it positively. How could something your body makes naturally be harmful?

In my research, as you look at the complications, the problems are found in the synthetic branch, and their mode of application. When you have an application that mimics the body's natural process, with an active, identical hormone, I have found no major negative effects. The synthetic progestins, such as MPA, have increased likelihoods of breast cancer. [ii]

The bottom line? *We want **in** our bodies what is natural **to** our bodies.*

Let's Begin the Conversation

I've laid out this book like a conversation. Imagine coming into my office and sitting down. You have my undivided attention. And you've come prepared with a list of questions about Bio-identical Hormone treatment.

That's the way I've structured this book. I've taken the most often-asked questions and given honest, straight-forward answers.

I'll show you the problem of decreasing hormone levels and how they affect us physically. You will see that when our hormone levels return to normal – to where they should be – your body will be strengthened and you will have the best chance to age gracefully and stay healthy and strong.

I will show you how hormones work. I will discuss six causes for lower hormone levels today; and I'll delve into some of the medical studies and literature that show the benefits received from proper hormone treatment.

I will detail the difference between synthetic hormone treatments (and its dangers) and bio-identical hormone treatment (and its benefits). We will see that BHRT replaces deficient hormones, repairs our bodies on a cellular level, restoring health, and ultimately revitalizing our overall well-being.

I will discuss the process of BHRT treatment and talk about how to get started at *The Youth Institute.*

I have included a short bibliography, listing five foundational books that I believe you will find helpful as you do your own investigation.

Ready to get started? Let's get back to the basics and get your life back!

Greg Brannon, M.D. and *The Youth Institute*

Chapter 1 – Is This Normal?

A ging is inevitable. The medical community and today's society have accepted this. We are constantly reminded that the following are normal or common occurrences because of aging:

- It is common to have a decreased libido as we age.
- It is common for women to lose interest sexually, to suffer from vaginal dryness, and to experience unexplained mood swings.
- It is common for women to have PMS, hot flashes, and night sweats.
- It is common that our current population has an ever-increasing number of people being diagnosed with dementia, Alzheimer's, and diabetes.
- It is common to experience significant weight gain as you age and to have difficulty losing that weight, no matter how much you diet or exercise.
- It is common for men to have an absence of nighttime erections and to have difficulty maintaining a strong erection during intercourse.
- It is common for men to lose muscle mass, muscle tone, and to experience weight gain, especially around the waist.
- It is common for young couples, 25-28 years of age, to only have sexual intimacy once or twice a quarter.
- It is common for young people to be on three or four anti-depressants at a time.

These things have become acceptable and it is a shame that we as a society do not question these occurrences. They are common but they are not normal.

Common is not synonymous with normal.

The good news is that they can be addressed and remedied.

Over the last five decades, our society has seen an alarming increase in the onslaught and intensity of diseases that we have accepted as normal. We have a generation of adults that are suffering in great numbers from diseases that previous generation minimally experienced. Fifty years ago, diseases such as diabetes, dementia and Alzheimer's were far less prevalent. In the past 50 years, cardiovascular disease has skyrocketed. Diseases such as diabetes, dementia and Alzheimer's were far less prevalent. Now those diseases are all too common.

But here is the key: ***common does not mean normal.***

I define ***normal*** to mean *"the way we were designed."* Just because many people are experiencing those symptoms doesn't mean that is the way we were designed.

> ***"Common" does not mean "normal."***

Have you ever stopped to consider that *"getting older"* does not have to mean *"falling apart"*?

Why does this happen? What's going on with your body?

We Lose Hormones as We Age

Every one of us longs for health and vitality. And yet it is common for men and women to experience decreasing hormone levels as they age, resulting (among other things) in decreased energy and focus.

When scientists were seeking to harness nuclear energy, they realized if they fired a neutron of uranium against other uranium atoms, they could create an unbelievably powerful nuclear reaction. This was the method used to create the ^{235}atomic bomb. The neutrons released when the atoms split would, in turn, strike and split other ^{235}U atoms.

Think about that. Scientists discovered – and harnessed – a power source of energy (sometimes used for good, sometimes for evil) that was revolutionary.

This same type of reaction happens in your body and mine.

Testosterone starts a chain reaction in our body. It replenishes our cells, which in turn affect our organs and systems throughout our whole body.

Through bio-identical hormone replacement therapy (BHRT), science has identified an effective and safe way to replenish the power source (hormones) in our bodies.

Did you get that?

No longer must we be resigned to living with the debilitating effects of low hormones. No longer do we have to suffer from diseases without having the natural resources and power to fight those diseases. It is a revolutionary concept that has changed the lives of thousands of people. And it can change yours. It can help you get your life back.

But please note …

BHRT is not a panacea. It is not a magic wand that can be waived over your body so you will never be sick again. But when your hormone levels return to normal – to where they *should be* – your body will be strengthened, and you will have the best chance to age gracefully, and stay healthy and strong.

I am going to be very practical. I want to answer the questions you are asking. I will delve into the science behind bio-identical hormone replacement therapy only to the extent that it helps answer the questions you have. Visit our website to find extensive resources and scientific research papers. Go to www.TheYouthInstitute.com to find hundreds of articles and the latest in medical research.

> *When your hormone levels return to normal – to where they should be – your body will be strengthened and you will have the best chance to age gracefully and stay healthy and strong.*

Question

What happens when my hormone levels are out of balance?

First, let me put my OB/GYN hat on and talk first to the women, specifically about changes in their levels of testosterone, estrogen, and progesterone.

Women

Changes in Testosterone

Women need testosterone – it's not just a men's hormone! Testosterone levels in twenty-year old women are typically between 70-90 ng/dL. What I am seeing in today's women are ranges much lower: between 8 and 30. When those women reach the age of fifty, I see their levels drop more significantly, to between 2-10 ng/dL. On the average, women lose 3% of their testosterone each year. By menopause, women have lost 70-90% of their total testosterone.

What does this mean? It means as a woman, you are losing all of the benefits of having an optimal level of testosterone in your brain, heart, and throughout your body.

Tang detailed a study where Alzheimer's patients were given testosterone treatments. Though there is no cure for Alzheimer's, Tang showed how the disease was slowed and had some regression and some very positive outcomes after participants in the study were given the testosterone treatments. [iii] Other studies confirm these benefits. [iv]

Women need testosterone!

The human body is like a finely-tuned engine. It converts cholesterol to hormones that are necessary for optimal functioning. This diagram shows the pathway from cholesterol to progesterone to testosterone to estrogen.

Method of Enzymatic Breakdown of Testosterone (*Diagram*):

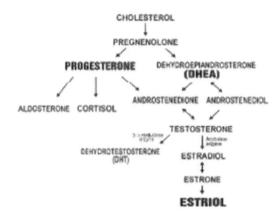

Changes in Estrogen

Estrogen is produced during the menstrual cycle as the result of ovulation. Menstruating women produce estrogen from the time their periods start as teenagers until menopause. Levels can fluctuate from 50-400 pg/ml. At menopause, a woman's body stops producing estrogen and her levels of estrogen drop to zero.

This may lead to a variety of symptoms, including:

- PMS, irregular menstrual cycle, heavy bleeding

- weight gain

- decreased sex drive, mood swings, and depression

- thyroid dysfunction

- fibroids, endometriosis

- gallbladder problems

- breast tenderness, fibrocystic breasts

Changes in Progesterone

Progesterone, testosterone and estradiol are all made in the ovaries. During a woman's monthly cycle, progesterone peaks after ovulation, a time when most women seem to feel their best.

> *At menopause, a woman's body stops producing estrogen and her levels of estrogen drop to zero.*

Levels of progesterone begin to decline, commonly by age thirty-five. At this time, you may notice changes in your periods, such as prolonged bleeding and/or shorter times between menstrual cycles. You may also experience mood swings and have more trouble sleeping.

It is at this point that many women complain to their doctors about anxiety, sleeping problems, and depression. That is why progesterone can be thought of as the anti-stress hormone.

In the chart below, you will see graphed changes in the levels of estrogen and progesterone throughout a women's menstrual cycle. But where are the testosterone levels in this diagram? Graphically speaking, they would be way at the top of the page. What is the reason for this? Remember this equation:

"T" = 10 x "E"

In other words, the T is the Testosterone level and the E is the Estrogen level. The Testosterone level is ten times the Estrogen level.

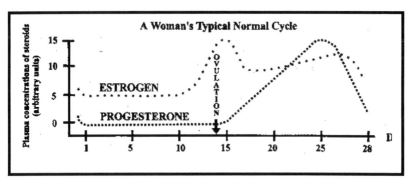

A woman's menstrual cycle affects her hormone levels

Women, the important aspects to note here are:

- The menstrual cycle occurs in two phases. The beginning of the cycle is known as the follicular phase and the final part of the cycle is considered the luteal phase. Midway through the cycle, between days twelve and sixteen, is when ovulation occurs.

- The levels of estrogen and progesterone fluctuate consistently through every menstrual cycle.

- It is when you know how a normal menstrual cycle works that you are able to understand the symptoms of premenstrual syndrome (PMS), perimenopause, and menopause. These symptoms are often the result of hormone imbalance.

- An irregular menstrual cycle is a good indicator of hormonal imbalance.

When a woman's hormone levels drop, she will begin to enter into menopause where common symptoms include:

- *Menstrual periods that occur less frequently and eventually cease*

- *Heart pounding or racing*
- *Hot flashes (usually worst during the first one or two years)*
- *Night sweats*
- *Skin flushing*
- *Problems sleeping (insomnia)*
- *Decreased interest in sex or changes in sexual response*
- *Forgetfulness*
- *Headaches*
- *Mood swings including irritability, depression, and anxiety*
- *Urine leakage*
- *Vaginal dryness and painful sexual intercourse*
- *Vaginal infections*
- *Joint aches and pains*
- *Irregular heartbeats (palpitations)*

Can you relate to some or all of these?

Lab tests can be performed to look for changes in hormone levels. Test results can help determine if you are close to or have already gone through menopause. Lab tests may include Estradiol, Follicle-stimulating hormone (FSH), and Luteinizing hormone (LH).

Men

Now, let me speak to the men. As a man ages, his hormone levels drop as well. Optimal testosterone levels are between 800 and 1,200. But I see men come into my office every day with levels in the 100s and 200s. Typically I see men's hormone levels decline every year as they age.

Natural testosterone not only helps a fifty-year-old man feel like he is thirty again, it protects his overall health.

You will notice on the chart below that men's testosterone levels historically decrease as they age.

Natural testosterone not only helps a fifty-year-old man feel like he is thirty again, it protects his overall health.

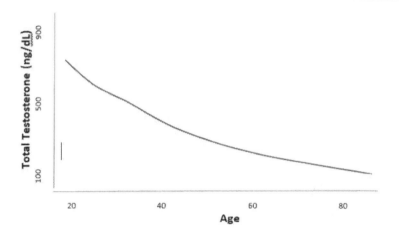

This graph should alert us to the changes that are happening in our bodies. Something is different. And that difference has dramatic effects.

Question
What does all this mean to men and women?

Think of your body as an engine. In your twenties, that engine was firing away on all eight cylinders. You had energy, focus and concentration, sexual drive, muscle-mass and great memory. You were a warrior!

But something started happening around age forty. At first the change was almost imperceptible. But soon, you began noticing that you could not do the things you used to. You became irritable, anxious. Things were "different" sexually. That once-powerful eight-cylinder engine was now down to three or four cylinders ... and you could feel the effects. By the way, these "engine problems" are something previous generations did not experience ... at least to the levels we are seeing them today.

The Effects on Women and Men

There are many signs and symptoms of testosterone and estrogen deficiency in women. For women, things start changing as they age. And because of that, numerous women begin experiencing some or many of the following symptoms:

- *Hot flashes*
- *Anxiety*
- *Irritability*
- *Fatigue*
- *Loss of energy*
- *Poor focus*
- *Poor concentration*
- *Depression*
- *Night sweats*
- *Vaginal dryness*

- *Fibromyalgia*
- *Osteoporosis*
- *Decrease in sexual interest*
- *Restless leg syndrome*
- *Painful intercourse*
- *Higher bad cholesterol*
- *Arthritis*
- *Alzheimer's*
- *Weight gain (despite exercising)*
- *Loss of memory*
- *A general loss of muscle tone.*

For men, the effects of testosterone deficiency can include some or many of the following:

- *Anxiety*
- *Irritability*
- *Fatigue*
- *Loss of energy*
- *Poor focus*
- *Poor concentration*
- *Decreased nocturnal erections*
- *Arthritis*
- *Loss of concentration*
- *Elevated lipids (cholesterol and/or triglycerides)*
- *Heart attack*
- *Stroke*
- *Decreased sex drive and erectile dysfunction*
- *Lack of ability maintain a hard erection*
- *Fatigue*

- *Loss of muscle mass and tone*
- *Diabetes*
- *Hypertension*
- *Weight gain around the waist*
- *Weight gain in spite of exercise*
- *Loss of confidence*
- *Depression*

Is any of that **normal?** **NO!** It might be *common,* but it is not *normal.* It is not the way God designed our bodies to age.

We are all designed to *age gracefully* and to be on top of life. Women, you don't need to dread *"the change of life"* time. Men, you can still be the warriors you were created to be … long into your seventies and eighties.

But something is wrong … and we know it.

It's No Longer Just an "Aging" Issue

Unfortunately, there is more to this sad story. I am seeing something at *The Youth Institute* that I never thought I would see. Young men – men in their late teens and twenties – are coming into my office with testosterone levels dangerously low, in the 100s and sometimes below that.

Some of these men are returning from serving our country in military service in Afghanistan and Iraq. Others are in college or just starting their careers.

They are depressed, lethargic, and sometimes suicidal. They have lost sexual interest and have changed from the *"warriors"* they once were to being complacent couch-potatoes.

Derek's Story

Derek [v] came into my office at his mother's request. She knew some friends who were patients of mine who had seen encouraging and positive results through BHRT.

As a twenty-two-year-old, Derek had struggled for years with depression, anxiety, fear, insecurity and inferiority. Despite treatment from doctors and psychiatrists, his symptoms were only getting worse. A top high-school athlete, he was now sedentary and lethargic, and his grades dropped to rock bottom. And he began to contemplate suicide.

After running the appropriate lab tests, and seeing his need, I put him on our *Youth Institute* BHRT treatment. In Derek's own words, he sensed no change after two weeks. After four weeks, still there was no discernable improvement.

But six weeks to the day after beginning treatment, he woke up that morning and *"everything was different."* His depression lifted. His focus returned. His hormone levels rose to a normal level, and Derek had his life back again.

> **"It was like someone flipped a switch and the lights came back on!"**

He remarked, *"It was like someone flipped a switch and the lights came back on!"* He has now returned to playing college lacrosse and excelling in school.

Question
Why did this dramatic change happen?

Derek's health and well-being returned when we put the body back in balance. He went back to normal. His hormones returned to their true normal level – and he is experiencing the difference. Simply put, at *The Youth Institute,* **the NEW YOU is the OLD YOU!**

> ## The NEW YOU is the OLD YOU!

My heart goes out to the thousands of Dereks out there who are suffering from testosterone deficiency and have lost hope. My heart breaks for men and women in their 40s, 50s, 60s, and even into their 70s who have been told, *"You're just going to have to live with these changes to your body."* Yes, something is wrong ... and you deserve to hear the truth. And I believe with all my heart that the truth will set you free.

There Is Hope!

Fortunately, there are answers. There is hope.

I believe in liberty and freedom. I believe in those principles with all my heart. I believe in our constitutional form of government that protects personal liberty. We have the right to be free.

That includes being free as it relates to our health. We must be free to take our health-matters into our own hands.

Moving forward, I am going to honestly and forthrightly answer your top questions about Bio-identical Hormone Replacement Therapy.

- You will understand how hormones work in your body and why you need them to be at optimal levels.

- You will discover the critical and life-changing difference between synthetic hormones that Big Pharma is pushing today, as opposed to natural and safe bio-identical hormones.

- You will learn how BHRT will return your hormone levels to normal, how it will restore health and vitality, and how those normal hormone levels will help keep your body healthy and guard against various diseases.

- You will read about *The Youth Institute's* pellet solution and procedure, and discover why this is the premier solution out there for BHRT treatment.

- You will find the next steps for BHRT pellet treatment and how to get started at *The Youth Institute.*

Let's get your life back!

Arrogance and Ignorance

I am so excited about BHRT – and to tell you about this treatment. This is what has caused me to enter a second career medically. I had been in an OB/GYN practice for 26 years. During that time, I prescribed synthetic hormones for women entering menopause. I didn't know any better. It's what I had been taught in medical school, residency, and post-residency training. I was taught that there was no difference between the way synthetic hormones and bio-identical hormones work in our bodies. Boy, was I wrong!

About ten years ago, I was introduced to Bio-identical Hormone Replacement Therapy through a friend who had started the treatment himself. My first reaction was to say, *"Hey buddy, you're going to kill yourself. That stuff causes prostate cancer!"*

To be honest, it was my own arrogance that caused me to be closed minded on this issue. My arrogance as a medical doctor led to ignorance about BHRT.

My arrogance led to my ignorance!

Fortunately, I've always been a science-nerd. I've always read and studied. And the changes in my friend's life intrigued me ... so I began doing my own research and study.

I not only came to the conclusion that BHRT was essential and effective ... I became a patient as well. I know first-hand the results of this treatment. I believe in it with all my heart – and I'm going to share it with you.

Liberty and Freedom

We were designed to experience liberty and freedom – politically, relationally, and medically. I close this chapter with a quote from one of our Founding Fathers, Thomas Jefferson:

"If people let the government decide what foods they eat and what medicines they take, their bodies will soon be in as sorry a state as are the souls of those who live under tyranny."

Greg Brannon, M.D. and *The Youth Institute*

Chapter 2 – How Do Hormones Work?

Our bodies are unique and wonderfully designed. They have been created to function in hormonal balance. When our bodies experience that balance, the result is health and fitness. But when our hormones are out of balance, the results can be disastrous, as we saw in the previous chapter.

Question
How do hormones work?

Hormones are chemical messengers created in the body to transfer information from one set of cells to another. As they are released into the bloodstream, they coordinate and control the various functions of the body to maintain health and stability.

The endocrine system in your body is made up of glands that produce and secrete these hormones to regulate the activity of cells or organs. Hormones regulate the body's growth, metabolism, sexual development and function. When our hormone levels drop, and become out of balance, our health is affected.

Testosterone is the chemical that enables every single cell in your body make protein. This DNA cell replication is called *transcription.* What are you made up of? Cells and cellular structures. When your cells are weak, your organs and systems are weak, and you are weak.

Hormones are designed to strengthen our bodies at the cellular level. Therefore, we must get to the root causes to find out what goes wrong when hormone levels drop.

> *Hormones are designed to strengthen our bodies at the cellular level.*

Let's talk a little science for a moment ...

As our bodies grow and develop, carefully orchestrated chemical reactions activate and deactivate parts of our bodies such as our cardiovascular system, our nervous system, and our immune system. *Epigenetics* is the study of changes in our bodies caused by chemical reactions and the factors that influence our DNA structure. That structure can be affected by environmental factors, diet, viruses, and even vaccines.

You might not feel the effects of these changes initially. At first, they might be imperceptible. But given enough time, these changes will show up.

Travison's 2007 paper [vi] details how testosterone levels have decreased every decade for the last sixty years. Why is this? The number one reason is due to endocrine-disrupting chemicals (estrogen mimickers). These chemicals influence the structure of steroids (or sex hormones) in our body. Please note: the term *"sex hormones"* does not mean *sex.* "Sex hormones" are the structures in our body composition, much like a brick house is made out of *bricks.* A backbone of the 27-carbon structure in your body is *cholesterol.* From that cholesterol is formed your *cortisol,* your *testosterone,* your *estrogen,* your *progesterone,* and all the precursors to that.

When these endocrine-disrupting chemicals spread, our structure is compromised. Why? These estrogen mimickers are located at all the pathways in our bodies. They affect your overall physiology – from the hypothalamus to men's pituitary gland, your testes, ovaries, and adrenal glands.

What does this mean?

Let's go back to our brick house illustration. The smallest structure in our body is a cell. Cells group together to make up your internal organs. And those organs group together to make up systems in your body.

A brick house is made of ... bricks! But you need something to hold the bricks together. If you simply stack those bricks together, one on top of another, to form a wall, it will be a very unstable wall. Bricks need mortar to hold them together. The bricks are strong, only to the extent where they are working together.

What mortar does for bricks, hormones do for the cells. It strengthens them and helps them function efficiently and effectively.

> *Hormones strengthen our cells and help them function efficiently and effectively.*

Question

What is causing my hormone levels to drop?

There is a myriad of causes. **First,** the cause may be environ-mental. For example, there are phthalates (plasticizers) that are found in polyvinyl chloride (think: PVC piping) that is prevalent in your home. When the PVC piping begins to break down, those foreign substances are released into the water supply and find their way into your body. This is the most-potent endocrine-disruptor there is, as it interferes with the actual formation of testosterone in your body. Think about that: *all the water you drink and cook within your home goes through that PVC piping!*

This affects all of us, no matter what our age. For example, the *World Health Organization* (WHO) has seen testosterone levels in boys 6-12 years old decrease 24-34% in the last few years. The WHO calls this a *gender bender* that has caused obesity, Type 2 diabetes, infertility, dementia, and loss of memory. They are currently campaigning to get PVC piping outlawed in our country.

These phthalates have also been found in 100% of pregnant women, so they are actually affecting the baby in the womb. All of us suffer from these endocrine-disrupting chemicals.

There is a specific signal that programs cells in your body to die. It's totally normal and healthy for 50 billion cells in your body to die every day! But studies have shown that phthalates can trigger what's known as *"death-inducing signaling"* in testicular cells, making them die earlier than they should. [vii] As a man, that scares me! *"Studies have linked phthalates to hormone changes, lower sperm count, less mobile sperm, birth defects in the male reproductive system, obesity, diabetes and thyroid irregularities."* [viii]

Second, the cause may be the result of certain medicines we take. For example, studies have shown that 35-50% of men will experience a decrease in their testosterone levels when on statins. [ix]

What is a statin? Statins are a class of lipid-lowering medications. They are typically prescribed for those who have heart disease and high cholesterol.

Third, your diet and the foods you consume will affect your hormone levels. High-grain diets are devastating. There is more sugar content in a bowl of oatmeal than in a root-beer float and a bag of Twizzlers combined. Large amounts of sugar consumption cause Type 2 diabetes. And those who suffer from that have a 57% decrease in their free testosterone levels.

We all know consuming large amounts of sugar is not good for us. Eating too much sugar causes a barrage of symptoms including weight gain, abdominal obesity, decreased HDL and increased LDL, elevated triglycerides, high blood pressure, and increased uric acid levels.

Fourth, BPA plastics are dangerous. BPA stands for bisphenol A. It is an industrial chemical that has been used to make certain plastics and resins since the 1960s. They are often used in containers that store food and beverages, such as water bottles. I would encourage you to use BPA-free products, to avoid micro-waving plastics or putting them in the dishwasher, where the plastic may break down over time and allow BPA to leach into your foods.

Fifth, lack of sleep can cause testosterone levels to plummet. Our bodies were designed to need consistent, quality sleep. When you don't sleep well, it throws your body off. And one of the effects is a decrease in testosterone. When you are sleep-deficient, your body simply doesn't replenish testosterone naturally. This can actually be a vicious cycle, because we need testosterone to enter REM cycles and sleep well, but low levels of testosterone can also cause lack of sleep. We lose both ways!

Sixth and finally, various chemicals are dangerous. Everything from air fresheners to pesticides is potentially life-altering. A study in England found the chemical *atrazine* in -abundance at lakes near certain pharmaceutical plants. (*Atrazine* is an herbicide used by farmers to control destructive weeds.) And at those lakes, researchers noticed there were no more male frogs. They had all been converted to females during the embryo-genesis phase of their development.

And guess where much of that atrazine ends up? In our corn, sorghum, sugar cane, and other foods.

We are all exposed to these dangerous chemicals. We are all familiar with *Roundup.* Currently law suits are being filed against *Roundup's* maker, Monsanto, for a failure to warn farm workers and those in the forestry and landscaping industries of potential risks of cancer related to exposure to *Roundup.*

But guess what? It's not just those farm workers who have been exposed. Studies have shown that 97% of us will have traces of *Roundup* when we urinate. And when those life-altering chemicals get into our body, they wreak havoc on our system structure.

Chemicals such as aluminum and mercury are extremely dangerous to humans. Do you know the highest way to get those chemicals into our bodies? It is not *only* through the environment – but through simple vaccines as well.

We are the most vaccinated country in the world. But did you know that, despite all of our vaccines (or perhaps *because of all of our vaccines*) America is 43rd out of 43 Western civilized countries in infant mortality, fetal death, and first year death? Stop and think about why that is – and what may be the cause of all of these medical issues. *The Institute of Medicine* (IOM) now admits, *"Vaccines are not free from side effects, or 'adverse effects.'"*

One of the results of these endocrine-disrupting chemicals I see in many of my patients is low levels of Vitamin D. A paper recently came out of Germany linking "Low D" (Vitamin D) to "Low T" (testosterone).

Exposure to fluoride is a controversial topic, because fluoride is everywhere. It is not only a common ingredient in toothpaste, but many cities add fluoride to their water supply, to encourage oral health. Only sixteen countries in the world put fluoride in their water. The United States is one of them... and the results are shocking:

Fluoride has been shown to weaken skeletal health, causes arthritis, to be toxic to the thyroid, calcify the pineal gland, accelerate female puberty, harm male and female fertility, negatively affect kidney health, harm the cardiovascular system, and have negative effects

> *Warning: be aware of what is going into your body!*

on your mind and ability to think clearly. The number one reason for poison control calls concerning fluoride are for children who have eaten toothpaste. Warning: be aware of what is going into your body!

Whether it is cosmetics you apply to your face, or fake sugars that you add to your drink and food, you are exposing yourself to dangerous chemicals that previous generations never had to deal with.

Question
The Bottom Line: How can I function optimally?

Our bodies are unbelievable filters. We are designed to be able to battle all types of infections and diseases. We are designed to age gracefully and handle the challenges of growing older. But that requires **functioning optimally.**

The engine oil and filter in your car were designed to lubricate and protect parts from contaminants and wear. But over time, those elements become thin and no longer protect the way they used to.

Have you noticed how your car engine sounds differently when you start it after you have run it 4,000 miles on the same oil? You can tell something is *"not right."* Then you put fresh oil in and it returns to its optimum performance. Changing your car's oil every 4,000-6,000 miles is crucial to its health.

Your body functions the same way. Over time, hormone levels decrease. They must be renewed and restored.

The pellet replacement therapy you will read about in this book starts with an initial insertion. Each pellet insertion therapy lasts four-to-six months, until your hormone levels need another *"fill up."* Coming into *The Youth Institute* and receiving each treatment keeps our hormone levels at their optimal point and your body functioning at its best.

Bridgette's Story

Bridgette was an OB/GYN patient of mine. An athlete all of her life, she worked out and trained consistently. But when she reached her forties, she noticed that the pay-off was not what it used to be. It became more difficult for her to stay in shape. She was experiencing a combination of less results from working out, as well as increasing lethargy. She also had been suffering from debilitating migraine headaches for most of her life.

Bridgette had been following a pretty strict nutritional plan of fresh vegetables, good protein, rarely eating processed foods and very few grain products for many years. She exercised frequently, changing up her routine regularly, but still was simply not achieving the results that she used to see and feel. She was frustrated, trapped on the roller coaster of not sleeping right, working out more, yet not getting good results.

At one of her annual examination appointments, she shared these struggles with me. We began talking about hormone replacement therapy. Her initial response was to say she needed to research and study about what I was telling her. (By the way, I LOVE that type of response. I want my patients to think for themselves. I never want them to simply take my word as truth. I encourage everyone: read, study, research, speak with those who have gone through BHRT ... and come to conclusions for yourself.)

She started the treatment over the following months and saw much improvement in her sleeping, energy level, mood and workout results. The migraines that she was accustomed to feeling on a regular basis, were virtually gone. She rarely had to take her migraine medicine. Her body was recovering faster from workouts, her cardio endurance was increasing and she was getting stronger. Her emotional health had improved. She felt happier and more positive. She is in tune with when the pellets are wearing down, as many patients are, (usually at the 3-month mark) and knows when it is time for another treatment. She has completed two Spartan races in the last year and is in better shape now than she was 10 years ago.

Human Physiology 101

To understand the results of low hormone levels, it is necessary to comprehend some basic facts about human physiology and how hormones work.

The testosterone hormone was first isolated by researchers in the early 1930s. The first paper published on how a testosterone pellet works was in a British journal in 1935. Pellet therapy was approved in the US in 1939. That's almost eighty years ago! Bio-identical hormone replacement therapy through pellet insertion is not something new. It has been around a long time!

> *BHRT through pellet insertion is not something new. It has been around for 80 years!*

Question
How does my body work?

How does testosterone work? How does your body work? Your DNA is the blueprint to make structures. Structures are made out of protein.

Testosterone bypasses the cellular membrane and goes into the nucleus membrane, diffuses in there and actually bonds to the DNA to turn on the DNA groups that form proteins. **It is the gasoline that turns everything on in your body's engine.**

Testosterone converts into both estradiol and into DHT (which is ten times more potent than testosterone).

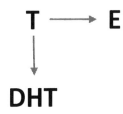

> **Testosterone is the gasoline that turns everything on in our body's engine.**

All three of these hormones enter the blood system and are distributed throughout our body.

The following diagram shows how hormones enter the blood stream and travel throughout your entire body. These *"chemical messengers"* travel throughout the body, coordinating complex processes like growth, metabolism, and fertility. The key point is to understand that hormones affect every cell in our bodies.

41

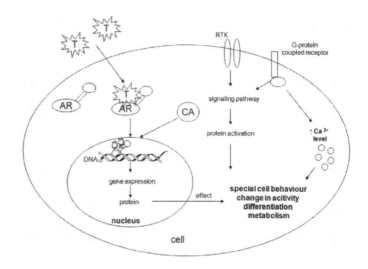

Question
What happens when my hormone levels are low?

When your hormones are low, that deficiency affects many parts of your body:

- You feel tired, drained, and short-on-energy to respond to many of the demands that life places on us.

- You are susceptible to depression and despair

- You are at greater risk of heart attacks, blood clots, strokes.

- You are more prone to dis-eases such as diabetes, dementia, and Alzheimer's.

- You are more prone to breast cancer, prostate cancer, and other types of cancer.

- Your sex drive and ability to perform sexually is lowered.

> *Testosterone is the gasoline that turns everything on in our body's engine.*

Testosterone levels for men are typically considered *"normal"* if they are anywhere from 301-1,197. That's a large range for normal! If I came to a sign in the road that signaled that there was a sharp curve ahead, but it said my acceptable speed could be anywhere from 30 mph to 70 mph, I'd be a little dubious.

Where should my hormone levels be as a man? Is 301 *"normal"* or is it a *"new average"* that I must be resigned to? It's the *new average*. It's not where your grandfather and my grandfather were at any age. But because of things we've been discussing, it is now the *new average*.

> **The "new average" doesn't need to be "new normal!"**

Here's the problem: *the new average doesn't help! It's not where your body needs to be!* **The new average doesn't need to be the new normal!**

Big Pharma and the insurance companies have re-defined what normal means. The "new normal," as insurance companies are trying to call it, doesn't help. It's simply a "new average" that lowers the bar but does nothing to improve our health.

Using that average range for male testosterone, a study of 858 Veterans over 4.3 years demonstrated that those in the bottom 25th percentile of testosterone levels had an 75% higher mortality rate.

Another study by Dr. Khaw published in the *Circulation* journal showed that men with testosterone levels of 350 or lower, compared with men who had levels of 564 or higher, had a 41% higher mortality rate. [x]

Clearly there are major effects when your levels are low. Our goal at *The Youth Institute* is to get your hormone levels back to where they should be – not where some doctors say is normal for *"your age"* – but where they really should be, so you can have the energy, health and vitality that you need.

You only have one body. You only have one life. How do you want to live it?

Question
What happens when my hormone levels return to where they should be?

It is amazing ... almost miraculous ... to see the difference in your body when testosterone levels return to the normal range. Research has shown that people with normal testosterone levels see:

- Less acute heart attacks

- Less blood clots

- Less strokes

- Less diabetes

- Less chance of dementia

- Less chance of Alzheimer's

- Less prone to depression

- Less cancer

- More energy

- More sex drive

- Greater ability to think clearly

Look through that list. And ask yourself, *"Who wouldn't want that?"* I sure do. And those are the results I've seen in the lives of my patients at *The Youth Institute* for the last five years.

Question
Are there medical studies and literature that I can read to back up these facts?

I have on my computer and in my office 360,000 articles on hormone therapy and its benefits. Because of the size and nature of this book, I can only mention a few here. I am planning a future, larger, more medically-documented book that will be able to go in-depth in this area. But that is why we have many of these articles available on our web site and in our office. They are available for you. And I encourage you to study, to do your own research, and to investigate what modern researchers are finding.

These documented studies show the positive effects of hormone treatment on our cardiovascular system, and our nervous system, our metabolic system. They demonstrate how the overall effects of aging can slow down when your body is performing optimally. And they show the positive effects in our sex lives and sexual performance.

The Effects of Low Testosterone

Korenman found that half of healthy men between the ages of 50 and 70 years have a testosterone level below the lowest levels seen in healthy men aged 20 to 40 years old. [xi] That means men are seeing a 50% decrease in their testosterone levels as they age into their 50s to 70s. As I mentioned earlier, Travison's research goes back sixty years showing a trend of decreasing testosterone that continues to this day.

Dr. Shores, writing in *The Archives of Internal Medicine* in 2006, described how a decrease in testosterone led to an eighty-eight percent increase in mortality compared to men with higher testosterone levels. [xii]

Hak's study in 2002 showed that when decreased levels of testosterone were present, there was an increased presence of arthrosclerosis. [xiii]

Dr. Morgentaler describes many of the "soft symptoms" that are hard to measure and even at times hard to describe. He calls it *"the loss of one's Mojo."* [xiv] I agree with him, because I've seen so many men come back to my office after testosterone treatment. They are sleeping better, focusing better, enjoying sex more, and having the energy and drive that they lacked before.

Cardiovascular Questions

Many of my patients have questions about their heart. There is a large misconception that cardiovascular patients get worse with hormone treatment. That has been proven false. In fact, the reality is just the opposite. English's study showed that treating angina patients with testosterone showed significant improvement. [xv]

Rosano's 1999 study looked at people who had exercise ischemia (where you get on the treadmill and work until your heart hurts). When they were on the treadmill and began experiencing symptoms such as shortness of breath and elevated heart rate, they were then given gel-testosterone. They were not given pellets because researchers wanted to be able to see if there was an instant effect. And they did ... patients saw an immediate improvement. [xvi]

> *Hormone replacement therapy is not only "not bad" ... it really helps!*

Then there is Pugh's study. The normal belief is that you don't give testosterone to people who have bad hearts. But Pugh came to the conclusion that increased levels of testosterone actually decreases the load on the heart. There were actually *positive* effects. In other words, giving testosterone had zero negative effects on the heart. [xvii]

My answer is that studies show that hormone replacement therapy is not only *"not bad" ... it really helps!*

Questions about Cancer

One of the concerns that many people have is that hormone treatment will increase their chances of cancer. Morley, in the January 2000 issue of the Mayo Clinic Proceedings, concluded *"There is no clinical evidence that the risk of either prostate cancer or benign prostate hypoplasia increases with testosterone placement therapy."* [xviii]

The Journal of the National Cancer Institute, 2008 detailed a collaborative study putting together seventeen independent studies and concluded, *"There is no association with increased risk of prostate cancer with increased testosterone or its by-products, DHT or estradiol."* [xix]

Dr. Abraham Morgentaler is a Harvard trained urologist and an internationally recognized expert in sexual medicine and male hormones. He wrote the phenomenal book *"Testosterone for Life."*

In that book, he addresses the common misconception that all hormone treatments are prone to cause cancer. He uncovered some fascinating facts. In his well-documented study, he went back to Huggins' paper in 1941. Huggins was the one who said treating with testosterone increased prostate cancer. Morgentaler went back to that paper, and he found that Huggins initially he did his study on dogs, not humans.

Huggins did a later study on only three humans. Two of the individuals were taken off the protocol in the middle of the study, leaving only one remaining person to follow. And that person had previously been castrated. Not exactly a great sample size! Nor was it a representative sample.

It is critical to realize that all of the subsequent literature referring to testosterone causing prostate cancer has gone back to this one study. [xx]

So how do we respond to the accusations that testosterone can cause cancer?

Morgentaler now has thousands of patients in his practice. From a twenty-year study written in the Journal of Urology, he described thirteen patients with proven prostate cancer (biopsied). Two-and-a-half years later, after treating them with testosterone, he biopsied them again. Fifty-four percent of those patients had no residual cancer (it was gone) and of the other 46%, none of them have had increased progression or metastasis of their cancer.

His conclusion was that when you HAVE cancer, you are actually decreasing the risk of cancer by treating with testosterone! And at the same time, you are also decreasing other risks, such as cardiovascular disease and dementia.

His conclusion?

"There is not now, nor has there ever been, a scientific basis for the belief that testosterone causes prostate cancer to grow." [xxi]

Osteoporosis

One of the most widespread and crippling diseases is osteoporosis. Worldwide, osteoporosis causes more than 8.9 million fractures annually, resulting in an osteoporotic fracture every 3 seconds. [xxii] Do we want to call this a new normal now? NO! It might be a new average – but it is unacceptable.

Osteoporosis is estimated to affect 200 million women worldwide - approximately one-tenth of women aged 60, one-fifth of women aged 70, two-fifths of women aged eighty and two-thirds of women aged ninety. [xxiii] It affects an estimated 75 million people in Europe, USA and Japan. [xxiv] For the year 2000, there were an estimated 9 million new osteoporotic fractures, of which 1.6 million were at the hip, 1.7 million were at the forearm and 1.4 million were clinical vertebral fractures.

Europe and the Americas accounted for 51% of all these fractures, while most of the remainder occurred in the Western Pacific region and Southeast Asia. [xxv] Worldwide, one in three women over age fifty will experience osteoporotic fractures, as will one in five men aged over fifty. [xxvi] It's a big problem.

So, what can we do? How can you take charge of your health to insure you have the greatest chance of success in keeping your bone structure strong?

Hormone treatment has been proven to significantly increase bone density. But it matters what type of hormone treatment you use. The American Journal OB/GYN has demonstrated the four-fold increase in bone density with bio-identical hormones over oral estrogen and 2.5 times greater than hormone patches. The details of those increases are:

- 1-2% per year for oral estrogen

- 3.5% per year for patches

- 8.3% per year for pellet therapy [xxvii]

Pellet BHRT has been shown to significantly increase bone density and to lessen the threat of osteoporosis.

This is just some of the evidence that is available in 360,000 articles and studies in medical journals. The weight of the evidence is overwhelming.

Again, I encourage you to do your own study and research. I believe you will come to the same strong conclusions I have about the effectiveness of hormone replacement therapy.

In the next chapter, we will look at two vastly different methods of treatment that are available today: *synthetic hormone replacement* and *bio-identical hormone replacement.* And we will see that BHRT is the safest and most effective hormone therapy available.

Chapter 3 – What's the Difference?

I had a patient ask me the other day, *"Why is it that, all of a sudden, I am seeing ads everywhere on television, in drug stores, and in magazines, advertising "hormone replacement therapy" and "testosterone boosters"? Those advertisements – and these therapies – weren't around when I was a kid. Why now? Was it just me not noticing them, or is this truly a new problem or even a fad?*

"And the lingo is confusing. Not only do I hear about "hormone replacement therapy," but now I'm seeing ads for "bio-identical hormone replacement therapy." What's this? Is it the same thing, but just "organic?" I'm confused. What's the difference?"

Those are good questions … questions that I have received from thousands of clients I've seen over the past five years. With a background in obstetrics and gynecology, I want both women and men to experience health and vigor, and to age gracefully.

As I said earlier in the book, after I recovered from my arrogance and pride, I began investigating these topics. I discovered how, with the right hormone treatment, we can achieve that younger, stronger, more energetic, and sexier reality.

But it must be the right treatment … with the right hormones.

When it comes to replenishing hormone levels in our bodies, doctors today have two options to choose from: *synthetic hormone replacement,* and *bio-identical hormone replacement.*

Let's look at the differences between these two methods of treatment, the benefits and dangers of each, and come to a reasoned conclusion about which is best for both men and women today.

Two quick points by way of introduction:

First, if your body sees something and it does not know how to metabolize or break it down, that's what causes the problems. Synthetic hormones, as we will see, do not come from the human body. They are foreign to it.

Second, those who tout synthetic hormones (and the ads are all over television) tell us that they are *"bio-equivalent."* That, my friends, is a play on words. It's also a lie, because bio-equivalent is not equal to bio-identical. They are very different!

> ***Bio-equivalent is not equal to bio-identical. They are very different!***

Question
What is Synthetic Hormone Replacement Therapy?

For years, doctors have typically prescribed synthetic hormone treatment for women who were menopausal. The two most common hormones they prescribe are *Premarin* and *Provera.* With the best of intentions, these drugs were given to women who were experiencing menopausal symptoms such as hot flashes, night sweats, hair loss, poor sleep, anxiety, and depression.

It is important to realize that these chemicals are not **natural**. They are chemical compounds that are foreign to the human body. And, as we will see, there are some very dangerous side-effects.

Premarin is a conjugated equine estrogen (CEE) that comes from … get this … horse urine. More specifically, this conjugated estrogen comes from the urine of a pregnant horse.

Women, do you really want something made from horse urine in your body?

Think about that for a moment: *does it make sense to use a chemical structure that is completely foreign to our make-up?* This hormone changes the normal ratio of estrogen in the body from 2:1 to 1:2 (the ratio of Estradiol to Estrone).

Provera is another synthetic chemical foreign to a woman's body. These tablets contain medroxyprogesterone acetate, which is a chemical derivative of progesterone.

When you take a drug that the body recognizes as foreign, there are side effects. When a body sees something that is foreign to it, and it cannot break that substance down, it attacks it.

Question
What are the dangers with Synthetic Hormone Replacement Therapy?

Some of the dangers and common side effects from women taking *Premarin* include:

- Increased risk of breast cancer

- Blood clots

- Fluid retention

- High blood pressure

- Headaches

- Leg cramps

- Increased risk of stroke

- Gall stones

- Tenderness of the breasts

- Worsened uterine fibroids

- Increased risk of diabetes

- Worsened endometriosis

- Increased risk of endometrial cancer

- Impaired glucose tolerance

- Nausea

- Vomiting

Prempro (a pill combining both *Premarin* and *Provera*) has been shown to cause an increase in breast cancer by twenty-six percent after four years.

The *Women's Health Initiative Trial,* which ended in 2002, showed that these synthetic hormones cause breast cancer, heart attacks, strokes, dementia, and blood clots.

In 2004, the results of *The Women's Health Initiative Memory Study* were released. This study conclusively proved that not only was

Prempro (the combination drug of *Premarin* and *Provera*) failing to protect women from declining mental capacity, it actually doubled the risk of dementia for women who took these drugs.

A 2005 study in France looked at 54,000 women who were treated with synthetic hormones. Those who were given bio-identical progesterone had 10% less breast cancer. Those who were treated with synthetic progesterone had a 69% increase in breast cancer. A 2007 follow-up study with 80,000 patients saw similar numbers. Another article concluded, *"The benefits of bio-identical estrogen on the heart were turned off by taking synthetic progesterone."* [xxviii]

Here's my question: *why would you want to do that to your body?* Why would you want to ingest any foreign substance (especially horse urine) into your body when there are better, more effective, and healthier alternatives?

> **Why would you want to do that to your body?**

Now, if you are a horse suffering from hormone imbalance, then *Premarin* might be just what you need. But if you aren't, I strongly encourage you to stay away from it ... or any of its derivatives.

One of my OB/GYN patients came to see me in my office recently, dissatisfied with the *Premarin* she was on, and scared of the side effects she was reading about. Her initial reaction was to get off hormones completely, but she knew the results of that would make her feel worse.

We talked for a while, and as I described the alternative of bio-identical hormone treatment, she lit up with excitement. Was it possible that there could be a solution that was both safe and effective?

Within two months of starting treatment, Jan returned to see me, elated with the results and relieved of her fears. *"I feel like I have my life back again."* She did … and without the dangerous side-effects of synthetic treatment.

Question
What are your best arguments against synthetic hormone replacement therapy?

In short, here is my case against the use of synthetic hormones in replacement therapy:

- These types of hormones are unnatural and foreign to the human body. Premarin uses a hormone from pregnant horse's urine that contains more potent estrogens than the human body can handle.

- The body has serious trouble assimilating these synthetic hormones and, in fact, will react against them. Conjugated estrogens must be processed in the liver before being distributed through the body. Taken orally, they must pass through the liver before entering the blood system – and that is where the problems occur.

  Why? Premarin has been known to elevate liver enzymes, causing a rise in clotting factors which increases the chances of clots in the veins and lungs.

When Pellet Bio-Identical Hormone Replacement Therapy is used, it completely by-passes the liver. Pellets are inserted into the fatty tissue of the buttocks, and dissolve directly into the blood system without ever going through the liver. In addition, bio-identical hormones are not nearly as potent as those conjugated estrogens from horses. Therefore, this danger is negated.

- The side effects listed above are dangerous and well-documented. Simply put, they cause more problems than they help.

- Synthetic hormones wind up treating symptoms, but do not get to the root of the problem.

Now, let's take a look at bio-identical hormones.

Question
What is Bio-identical Hormone Replacement Therapy?

There is a vast difference between synthetic hormones such as *Premarin* and *Provera* and bio-identical hormones. Bio-identical hormones are natural, using plant-based ingredients.

The Mayo Clinic has defined bioidentical hormones as *"compounds that have exactly the same chemical and molecular structure as hormones that are produced in the human body."* [xxix]

This means that the body recognizes bioidentical hormones as itself. This is critical. Traditional hormone replacement therapy uses drugs whose structure and nature are foreign to the human organism. Hormones, then, are not drugs. Hormones are molecules produced by our own glands and so do not come with the undesirable side effects of traditional hormone drugs—as long as the hormones prescribed are identical to those made by the body. [xxx]

Bio-identical hormones are plant-based and natural, as opposed to synthetic hormones, which are completely foreign to the human body.

The pellet that we use is made up of 99.5% natural testosterone that comes from yams. Their structure is *identical* to that of the human body. The other 0.5% of the pellet is composed of steric acid that allows the testosterone to hold together and to dissolve slowly when placed. This *identical-ness* is the *major differentiator* between bio-identical and synthetic hormones.

> *Bio-identical hormones are plant-based and natural, as opposed to synthetic hormones, which are completely foreign to the human body.*

This is important! It negates any chance of dangerous side effects. Because these hormones are *"bio-identical"* to your body's structure, your body will not reject it nor react against it. Unlike synthetic hormones that present dangerous consequences, BHRT is safe and effective.

Take a moment and read through the benefits of *BHRT* listed below. Does this sound like the positive health-model you have been looking for?

The Benefits of Bio-Identical Hormones	
Safe	Less prone to depression
Absorbed directly into blood stream	Less cancer
	More energy
Lowers chance of diabetes	More sex drive
Lowers Cholesterol	Less acute heart attacks
Lowers Obesity	Less blood clots
Increases clarity and cognitive ability	Less strokes
	Less dementia
Less prone to Alzheimer's	

What are the dangers of bio-identical hormones? It is the conclusion of doctors and researchers all around the world that bio-identical hormone replacement therapy is safe, proven, and effective.

Safe ... I have read extensively regarding the safety issue behind BHRT ... and I have never seen any research showing health risks. The research shows there are no major dangers in this treatment.

Proven ... Through our web site you have access to article after article that shows the proven results of BHRT.

Effective ... I've seen the results in thousands of lives through *The Youth Institute.*

> *Safe ...*
> *Proven ...*
> *Effective ...*
>
> *Those are the three words I would use to describe BHRT!*

Yes, there are some today who state that *all* hormone treatments can cause cancer. But as I said earlier, this conclusion is because these researchers have lumped all hormone treatments (synthetic and bio-identical) together. BHRT has become *"guilty by association."* However, I cannot find any research paper that shows a link to cancer with BHRT. The problems appear to be wholly centered around the *synthetic hormones* and their mode of application.

Let me make two other comments in regard to the chart on the previous page.

First, BHRT is not a cure-all. BHRT returns hormone levels to where they should be so your body can function the way *it* should. You will still age ... but now you will be able to age gracefully, the way you were designed. It is giving your body its best shot to cope with its environment.

Second, I was correct in stating there is no research that shows any life-threatening or long-term dangers from this therapy. However, there are some potential side-effects (minor ones, that are certainly non-life threatening) in certain patients of which I want all of my patients to be aware.

- The first side effect is that there can be a slight pain at insertion. In the next chapter, I will detail the simple and proven pellet insertion method I use. Here, I merely want to state there is "some" pain involved in the procedure. Typically, this pain lasts only a few seconds while injecting the lidocaine. The actual pellet insertion is painless, though you may feel slight pressure

  How much pain are we talking about here? Obviously, it differs from patient to patient, based on their pain-tolerance. Most patients say there was *"not much pain,"* or *"about as much as getting a blood draw."* In my experience, women have experienced less pain – mainly because they usually receive only one pellet at a time, where men can receive 3-10 pellets, depending on their lab levels. (Or could it simply be that men are wimps when it comes to experiencing pain?)

- The second side effect is that there is 2% possibility the pellet(s) will be expelled (for men). Nationally, this rate is significantly higher, closer to a 5-10% fall-out rate. But with the methods pellets *The Youth Institute* uses, we are seeing about a two percent expulsion rate. From my experience as a patient myself for over five years, I've had two pellets that were expelled. For women, pellet rejection is less than one in a thousand.

  So, what happens if that occurs? You simply call our office, come back in, and we will re-insert a replacement pellet.

- A small percentage of women (2-5%) have experienced some facial hair growth. Another small percentage of both men and women have experienced minimal amounts of hair loss. If either of these happen, there are steps that we can take to minimize this in the future.

- Finally, a small percentage of patients have experienced mild break-outs of acne. Again, this is treatable and not a long-term issue.

Let me re-emphasize: these side effects are mild. When you contrast them with the dangers that accompany synthetic hormone treatment (especially high cholesterol, obesity, heart attacks, strokes, dementia, and the other diseases that bio-identical hormones prevent), it is easy to see why so many people are choosing BHRT.

> *Incredible benefits, no dangers, mild and infrequent side effects.*

The bottom line: *incredible benefits, no dangers, mild and infrequent side effects.* What more do you want?

The case is clear. Bio-identical hormones are completely natural, definitely safer, and more effective than synthetic hormone treatment.

Question

What is the overall goal in Bio-identical Hormone Replacement Therapy?

The goal of BHRT is "to replace," "to repair," and "to restore."

It begins with *"replacing"* deficient hormones in your body and bringing them up to normal levels. When your testosterone levels are replenished, you restore vitality to each cell.

It continues with *"repairing."* Once those hormones are in your system and operating properly, they will act to bring health on the cellular level, then to the organs in your body, and then to the various systems in your body, such as our cardiovascular system. A replenished testosterone level is capable of defending against harmful elements to the body.

Finally, BHRT **"*restores*"** health and vitality to our entire body. When hormone levels are restored to normal, optimal levels, *"**health spreads."*** That's what I call **"revitalize."** So, the equation looks like this:

Replace ->

Repair ->

Restore =

Revitalize!

> *We simply get your body back to the basics.*

Bio-identical hormone replacement therapy simply gets your body back to the basics.

Mike's Story

No one can tell the story of *"health spreading"* better than Mike. I've known Mike for over twenty years. He was a friend and golfing buddy before he became a patient.

Mike is a former Big 10 quarterback at Northwestern. He could throw a football sixty to sixty-five yards. But this once stud-of-a-guy began to see his health deteriorate. He broke his right arm, ending his playing career, and had to have a cyst removed from his right hand the day before graduation. He never had the cyst on his left hand removed, and it continued to grow and spread, entrapping the nerves up his left arm to the point where his left arm was virtually paralyzed.

He graduated and went to his first job. Over the years, his arm condition got worse. His wife (a registered nurse) said, *"Your arm is getting deformed. It looks like a little alligator arm."*

Thirty years of pain took its toll. His arm was continually in lots of pain. His back, from years of football, hurt from stenosis in the neck and upper back. Doctors prescribed steroid shots to ease the pain, but one of those shots paralyzed Mike. He could not feel his lower extremities for several hours. They wheeled him into the emergency room where he eventually recovered. But no more steroid shots.

To compensate, the doctors started throwing pills at him. Little did he know that those pills further reduced his testosterone levels. That put him in a clinical depression, so they prescribed more pills. As late as a year ago, this once-great-athlete was talking with his doctor about going on disability. He was self-employed and could only work four hours a day, and maybe be productive only an hour a day. By his own admission, Mike was suffering from twenty of the twenty-five male low-testosterone symptoms we listed in chapter one. As he says, *"I was a mess physically, emotionally, spiritually, in all ways."*

Mike was one of my neighbors and one day we were talking about what was going on in his body. He was depressed and discouraged. To be honest, he was also desperate. As I told him about BHRT, it intrigued him. And he tried it.

Within weeks, his body started changing. Previously Mike had a gut … but soon he lost all his excess wait and the gut began to disappear. His muscles totally recovered and his back and arm pain went away.

Mike says, *"I'm not a doctor – I'm an engineer and a business man. I can't explain how all this happened. I just know the results. I was at the golf course the other day and a woman saw me and shouted out, "WOW! Those are the biggest biceps I've ever seen!" I looked around and said, "Who are you talking about?" All I can do is tell you that for me, it has been nothing short of life-changing. It has made every part of life better.*

He told me recently, *"Before I started BHRT, I was pale. Now I'm bronze again!"* Mike calls it *"Body by Brannon."*

Mike concluded, *"People wonder that with higher testosterone won't you be angrier? For me, I struggled with anger in those hard years. Now it's just different. I love harder. I live harder. And I enjoy life a whole lot more."*

Question
How does BHRT affect sexual libido and sexual performance?

That's a great question – and one that many of my patients (both men and women) are interested in. In fact, I know this is probably the section the guys turned to first!

Over the years, researchers have seen a direct correlation between BHRT and increased libido, sexual interest, sexual performance, and sexual fulfillment.

Carol's Story

Carol came to see me recently. Her husband was already a patient and had encouraged her to give BHRT a try. Carol had been on BHRT cream therapy for several years, but her hormone levels were still significantly low. She also had a major deficiency in her Vitamin D levels.

Within one week after placement, her sexual responsiveness and aggressiveness had returned. Needless to say, she and her husband are both *"satisfied customers."*

Kimberly's Story

Kimberly is a 49-year-old OB/GYN patient. I've known her for many years and delivered her babies. She started pellet therapy several years ago and came in for a check-up today. She said, *"Over the last two years, my husband and I have finally realized what our bodies are for. Even when we were younger, we only had sexual intercourse once or twice a month. Now we are having sex two-to-three times a week. It's been a great way for us to communicate and draw closer as a couple. You gave us our life back. You allowed me to know my body. The last several years have been phenomenal."*

Jake's Story

What about men? How does BHRT affect their sexual performance? Among other symptoms men often experience (see the complete list on page 13), Jake was suffering from erectile dysfunction. I could tell he was initially embarrassed to even bring this up to me in our consultation. I am very conscious to create a safe, open atmosphere during my consultations – and Jake responded with candor.

"I just can't get it up like I used to. I want to have sex with my wife, but I can't get hard enough."

Once we ran his labs, I pointed out to him where the problem was. And his response was, *"Doc, if it can fix this, I'm all in."*

Not only did Jake see significant improvement in his ability to have an erection, but there were also other areas where he saw change and positive results. His energy level and ability to wake up rested and refreshed were, in his words, *"back to what it used to be."* Jake was back to the basics.

Question
What studies do you have to show that BHRT is safer than synthetic hormones treatments?

Let's start with the women

Dr. Fournier's study was written up in *The Journal of Cancer 2005*. That study looked at 54,000 female patients. Half of the patients were treated with a combination of bio-identical estrogen and bio-identical progesterone. The other half was treated with a combination bio-identical estrogen and *synthetic* progesterone. The first group saw a decrease in breast cancer rates of 10%. The group that was treated with the synthetic progesterone saw an increased breast cancer rate 40%. xxxi

Two years later, Fournier looked at another 80,000 women over a longer period of time. Through that study, they saw zero breast cancer increase in the bio-identical group and 69% increase in the synthetic progesterone group.

Are there dangers for women that bio-identical hormone replacement therapy will cause cancer? ABSOLUTELY NOT!

What about for men?

Again, I refer you back to Dr. Morgentaler. He is a well-respected Harvard-trained urologist who is a national expert in these issues. After extensive studies and tests to determine if BHRT is cancer-causing in men, he has concluded, *"There is not now, nor has there ever been, a scientific basis for the belief that testosterone causes prostate cancer to grow."* [xxxii]

Question
What are your best arguments for *Bio-identical Hormone Replacement Therapy?*

The following points are my best-case for the use of bio-identical hormones in replacement therapy:

- There is an abundance of evidence that replacing lost hormones is essential to good health.

- Replacing low and declining hormones must be done with bio-identical hormones. This is the only kind of hormone that equates to the body's make-up and therefore is completely safe, without any of the negative side effects.

James' story

James came into my office having done his research. At our original consult, which often lasts 30-60 minutes, he was ready to sign up. His questions were all answered, and we ordered his labs. His testosterone level was 136, way below normal. Two days later, I performed his initial placement. I saw him at one of our public seminars about six weeks later and asked him how he was feeling. His labs now showed his T level to be over 1,100.

He said,

"Yesterday, I worked fourteen straight hours on three separate, highly intensive projects. I was able to keep up my focus, energy, and momentum throughout the day. My thinking was clear. My spirit was energized. And I was effective. I could not have done that six weeks ago. BHRT is really making a difference."

Do you know what my best argument for BHRT really is? The thousands of lives, like James, who have experienced these dramatic changes in their lives. That's my greatest privilege – to be a part of helping bring about that change! Our goal at *The Youth Institute* is simply to help make the new you the old you!

Greg Brannon, M.D. and *The Youth Institute*

Chapter 4 – What's the Process?

In one of our recent public seminars, Lindsay told her personal story of recovered hope. In her own words, she said:

"Twenty years ago, I had my first GYN appointment with Dr. Brannon. About four-and-a-half years ago, my husband and I felt that God was calling us to live and work in East Asia. The language there is one of the most difficult to learn, and my husband and I are both in our early 50s.

"About two years into our time there, we were teaching English to college students at a university in our city. They also wanted to involve us in playing ping-pong, badminton and other Asian games. I was post-menopausal and it was at that time I started thinking how little energy I had and how tired I was. I couldn't keep up with these students we were trying to minister to. In addition, my libido was low ... and six months before a return trip to the States, I also began experiencing pain during sexual intercourse.

"I am a registered nurse by trade, and I began looking on-line for help. Nothing was working ... and by the time we came back in the summer of 2015, I was in tears. At my annual check-up with Dr. Brannon, I shared with him what was going on.

"He looked at me and said, 'I have the answer.' And I replied, 'I knew you would!' He called me and my husband in to The Youth Institute and we had a consultation. I am very science-driven and my husband is very research-driven. We received the information and went home to do our own research and study. We looked every-thing up and came to the conclusion that this is what we needed to do.

*"We scheduled an appointment to have our pellets placed, and my first comment to Dr. Brannon was, 'You want to put **what, where**?' But because I had known him for over twenty years, I trusted him.*

*"On the pamphlet that Dr. Brannon gave us about the benefits of BHRT, the first benefit was **increased libido**. I will tell you that it was probably two to three weeks later, not even at the six-week mark, I started feeling like I was 29 years old again – not the 58 that I was. I was probably driving my husband crazy at that point!*

*"The second benefit on that pamphlet was **increased clarity**. My mom, who has since passed away, suffered from dementia and Alzheimer's for the last eight years of her life. I watched her suffer from the horrific effects of those diseases. Again, after several weeks of receiving the pellet placement, I could sense clarity and focus in my mind that I hadn't had in years.*

*"I also have seen **better cardiovascular benefits**. When we returned to East Asia, I found myself, unlike before, now being able to keep up with these college students. We need energy ... and that again is one of the greater benefits I've experienced."*

I hope by now I have convinced you of the effectiveness of bio-identical hormone replacement therapy. I trust that you are now ready to get started.

Question

Tell me more about the placement procedure.
What happens there?

The Youth Institute Pellet

We want the purest type of pellet possible. Over the years, we have worked with compounding pharmaceutical companies to produce the best and most effective pellet possible. To develop the pellet for men, we use organic yams as the precursor to the testosterone. The pellet is 99.5% pure yam-hormone. The other 0.5% is composed of steric acid acts as a lubricant, holding the pellet together in proper form. (It is important to note that this steric acid is not absorbed at all into your system.) We don't want the pellet to be too hard (other-wise, it won't dissolve) and we don't want it to be too soft (or it won't hold together). The ratio that we currently have is the best possible pellet for our purposes. Typically, a man will receive anywhere from 8-12 pellets at a time, depending on his lab levels. His pellet will contain bio-identical testosterone, with each pellet having a dosage of 1600-2200 mg of testosterone.

The pellet we use for women will contain both testosterone and estrogen. The dosage of the pellet will range from 75-125 mg of testosterone and 6-20 mg of estrogen.

Women are able to ingest oral progesterone, as it does not affect the liver.

So how do we do it? What about the placement of the pellets?

The Placement

Placing involves a simple stab incision into the fatty area of the buttocks. After cleaning the area with iodine and alcohol, I will numb you with 2% lidocaine solution.

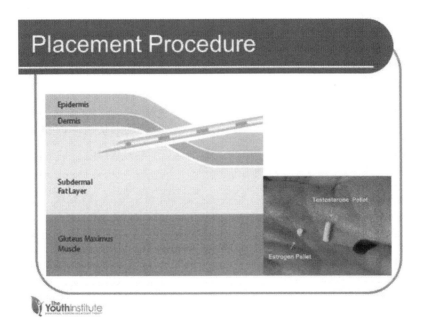

We then go in at a thirty-degree angle with a straw-like instrument to place the pellet(s) and then put a bandage and some tape over it to protect the area from infection.

Question
What are the chances a pellet can be expelled?

The Problem of Expulsion

The literature about this procedure will tell you that about 5-10% of the men may expel the pellet. For women, it is about one in a thousand.

It's really based on how hard the pellet is and how your body responds. That is one reason we have worked with highly regarded compound pharmacies to produce the pellet we use. Our expulsion rate is only 2% in men because of the makeup of the pellets. For women, it is one in a thousand.

Question

Now that I am ready to sign up, how do I become a patient at The Youth Institute?

First Steps

The first step is to call our office and set up an appointment for a consultation. There I will attempt to answer all your questions. We'll take as much time as necessary. (I also hold public seminars and, at times, the seminar can replace the initial consultation.)

We will then order your labs – you can have them done that day or whenever is convenient. Labs usually take 5-15 minutes, depending on their schedule that day, and I will have the report back on my desk in 24 hours.

At that point, we can schedule an appointment. I will prepare your personal treatment based on our *Youth Institute* algorithms. It usually takes 10-15 minutes to place the pellets and then you are good to go.

The Dosing Model

The dosing model is crucial. After doing this for the last five years, with thousands of placements, I've put together an algorithm based on each individual patient and their labs. Our algorithms have been developed over five years and are based on thousands of patients. We take your labs and design a dosage and treatment personally for you.

I hope you see immediate results and impact to your health and vitality in the short-term. But I went on BHRT for the long-term results and the benefits for things like arthrosclerosis, dementia, and diabetes. It's like taking vitamins every day. I don't see the short-term benefits, but I know I am building for long-term health. We jog, work out, and eat the right foods so that we're healthy now ... but especially as we age.

Dosage for Females

I want to make sure we have objective and subjective data. For pre-menopausal women, I am especially concerned with their testosterone levels. We will get them checked with the labs and make sure they are up to proper levels with treatment. Our staff at *The Youth Institute* will call you the next day to see how you are doing, and we will also re-check the labs in four-to-six weeks. We'll monitor how you feel (that's the subjective data) and also watch closely what the labs tell us (that's the objective data).

Also, once you have your initial consult with me, I will never charge again for another consult. What happens if you have questions the next week or the next month? Schedule an appointment. Come on in. I am here for you and to make sure all your questions are answered. Ask questions. Do your research. Bring articles to me that you've read. I want you to know more than I know. It's your body. Take charge of it.

Why is the subjective data so important? Because the best person to tell if this is working is *not* me telling you what the labs say (although that's important). The best person to tell if it is working is *you*. You'll know how you are feeling and what's going on inside of you. And the external, objective data will simply confirm that.

What BHRT treatment method is best?

What kind of bio-identical treatment is best? When you do pellet treatments, it mimics your ovary and testicle production identically. When you do a cream treatment, testosterone is not assimilated as strongly and the results are limited. When you do an oral treatment, you don't get enough dosage. And treatment through injections are outlawed for women. (They are available for men only, and even there, it results in levels that mimic a roller-coaster, with up-and-down spikes.)

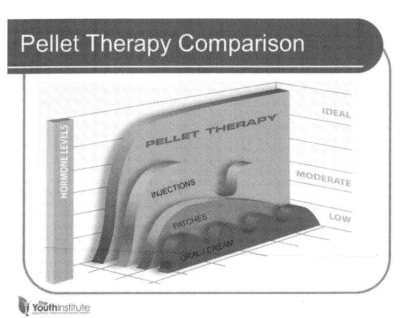

Pellet Therapy Comparison

Youthinstitute

Pellet treatment stays constant and goes directly into the blood stream. As you work out, your blood flow increases, and more testosterone flows through your system … just like it was designed to do. It mimics the way our body works.

As the pellet dissolves over time, you will want to get placed again after about four months. Why four, if the pellet is designed to last up to six months? Because you never want to "go low" again. Being placed again after four months keeps your levels constant.

For menopausal women, I want to replace estrogen. Our brains produce a chemical called FSH. I want to monitor both of those levels. What I look for specifically is when the levels go above 26 mIU/ml. The higher that number goes, the more you will sense symptoms like hot flashes, vaginal dryness, and sweats. So, as I monitor these numbers, I can watch for those symptoms.

As an OB/GYN, when I prescribed *Premarin,* I never got labs. I just gave the drug. There is no correlation between the dose of *Premarin* or the dose of *Estrace* and the lowering of their FSH level. It's like trying to fit a square peg in a round hole. That FSH level only goes down when the body recognizes the exact chemical it is supposed to recognize. ***That's the "round peg in the round hole."***

Progesterone is highest around post-ovulation times. Women tend to feel their best during the second half of their monthly cycle. We need to balance progesterone levels around those times. Progesterone levels can vary between 0 and 30 ng/ml … and I want to find the optimal levels for each woman.

Dosage for Men

I will also have labs run for all of my male patients. I am especially looking for their T level, which optimally should be over 800.

Often, I am finding men (even men in their twenties) who have such low testosterone (oftentimes in the 100s, sometimes even lower than that!) that it really concerns me. I will run their levels through our *Youth Institute* algorithm and come up with a dosage plan that includes the number of pellets they will receive. Once treated, we check back in 4-6 weeks with new lab tests – and invariably men's levels rise dramatically.

I want to find out who **you** are and what's best **for you.** That's why the subjective part is so important.

What about the long-term implications of this treatment? Some will raise the question of long-term dangers, when, in fact, the reality is just the opposite. A collaborative analysis published in the *Journal of the National Cancer Institute* om 2008 found that there was no association between the risk of prostate cancer and any hormone measured, including testosterone, DHT, estradiol, and others." [xxxiii]

When your body is optimally balanced, you will not be as susceptible to these other diseases. As I have said earlier, nothing is a panacea. But we all want our bodies to be functioning as efficiently as possible and as they were designed.

I asked Johanna to share her story of battling with an autoimmune disease.

Johanna's Story

"In March of 2014, I was diagnosed with an autoimmune disorder called Hashimoto's Thyroiditis. This condition causes a person's own body to attack the thyroid gland. The symptoms include joint pain, fatigue, brain fog, digestive issues, panic attacks, insomnia, heart palpitations, and weight changes. I had all of the above and went from a size 10 to a size 2 in the space of six months. I became very, very ill and had such debilitating joint pain that most of the time I could barely walk. At times, I needed to use crutches, and sometimes even a wheelchair. I was forced to quit my job. I was so sick that I went to live with my parents for several months. I saw thirty different doctors in one year, trying to figure out how to treat my condition.

"Unfortunately, conventional medicine is of little help when it comes to treating autoimmune disorders, which respond better to natural treatments than to drugs. Finally, I had the good fortune to find a Functional Medicine Practitioner who set me on a path to healing, using nutritional supplements and a Paleo diet. I have read and researched a tremendous amount, and I have been vigilant about sticking to the diet and taking the proper supplements. After two years, I am well on my way to putting my Hashimoto's into complete remission and am certain that I will be fully healthy and healed in the very near future.

"There were a few wonderful doctors who were instrumental in my recovery, and one of them is Dr. Greg Brannon. A problem that is common with Hashimoto's patients is hormone dysfunction, for which I tested positive. A significant part of the reason why I feel so much better is that Dr. Brannon was able to correct the erratic, abnormal fluctuations of my estrogen, progesterone, and testosterone. He did this not with dangerous synthetic hormones, but with all-natural bio-identical hormones which are made from wild yams and are actually good for your body. Bio-identical hormones, along with various other

helpful treatments, have taken away my pain and allowed me to heal. I am now walking well and my life is returning to normal.

"Dr. Brannon was incredibly supportive and possesses a wealth of knowledge. He gave me a book that changed my understanding of health care and how we can make ourselves healthy without drugs or surgery. Dr. Brannon inspired me to want to help other people to heal, as he has helped me. Even when I was at my lowest point, his words of encouragement confirmed that I was doing all the right things and gave me the will to persevere.

"At my most recent appointment with him, he was astounded at how well I was walking and how much progress I've made since the last time he saw me. I assured him that a huge part of my recovery had to do with the hormone treatments, and that I was so grateful for all he had done for me. He thanked me and said, "This is why I do what I do. Because the reward is so great when I can see a tremendous change in someone like you." He added, "You are a walking miracle, Johanna. Don't ever forget that. And don't ever give up your fight. You will heal yourself. Conventional medicine says you can't cure Hashimoto's, but they're wrong. You are living proof of that." I have thought of his words many times since and they always give me strength.

"Dr. Greg Brannon is a great man and a great doctor: educated, forward-thinking, compassionate and inspiring. I am lucky to be his patient, and I hope that more people like me will be able to benefit from BHRT."

Question

Will my insurance company cover BHRT?

You say, *"Dr. Brannon, I want to try this, but it costs money."* Yes, it does. But think about this: these treatments will actually benefit you for the rest of your life ... for today and into the future. Several dollars a day is a small price when compared to the cost of potentially life-threatening diseases later in life. Just ask Johanna if the cost was worth it!

Big Pharma is opposed to BHRT because they cannot make as much of a profit off it. Why? Bio-identical hormones are **natural**. As natural products, they cannot be patented. You cannot patent an organic molecule ... and therefore, pharmaceutical companies cannot make any money off it.

What about insurance? At this time, health insurance typically does not cover BHRT. I don't know about you, but I don't want the government telling me how or how not to take care of myself. I don't want a bureaucrat or an insurance company telling me what type of medications I should or shouldn't take. The most important property you own is you. **The one who cares the most about you is you.**

> *The most important property you own is you. The one who cares the most about you is you.*

I believe in personal liberty. And there is a freedom in taking personal responsibility for yourself.

Question

You've mentioned Vitamin D several times.
How does low D affect me?

There are numerous scientific studies regarding Vitamin D3, making it one of the most studied vitamins. There is no debate in the medical community that normal Vitamin D3 levels influence health.

At *The Youth Institute,* we monitor more than your hormone levels. We also track Vitamin D levels because we know that the process of getting you back to the basics involves all areas of your health.

What does Vitamin D3 do? [xxxiv]

- Vitamin D3 levels influence health.
- Vitamin D3 affects virtually every cell in your body and affects expression of around three thousand genes.
- It unlocks the genetic blueprints that are stored inside our cells.
- Vitamin D3 promotes healthy weight, blood sugar regulation, and blood pressure.
- It is involved in everything from bone strength and health to mood, immune function and optimal sleeping patterns.

Vitamin D3 can help with weight loss. According to a 2007 by the Women's Health Initiative, Calcium/Vitamin D3 slowed postmenopausal weight gain in women who were not getting enough calcium. We need Vitamin D to help the body absorb calcium and phosphorus from our diet. These minerals are also important for healthy bones and teeth. Anyone with Metabolic Syndrome, hypertension, pre-diabetes, and weight gain, should have their D levels checked and should be supplementing with Vitamin D to optimize their levels.

What are some symptoms of Vitamin D deficiency?

- Fatigue
- General muscle pain and weakness
- Joint pain
- Weight gain
- High blood pressure
- Restless sleep
- Poor concentration
- Headaches
- Bladder problems
- Constipation or diarrhea
- Depression

How can you find out if you are deficient in D3?

You need to have a blood test to check your Vitamin D levels. As part of your initial lab tests, we will also test your levels of Vitamin D. Once your level is determined, we will recommend your appropriate daily dose of supplementation.

The two main ways to get Vitamin D are by exposing your bare skin to sunlight, and by taking Vitamin D supplements. Most people do not get nearly enough sunlight due to their work schedules, lifestyle, and sunscreen use. The lack of UVB (ultraviolet B) does not allow our bodies to make enough Vitamin D.

I recommend supplementing Vitamin D3 with 5000 IU per day. This depends, of course, on your individual lab level. In addition to protecting you from the Vitamin D-Deficiency symptoms listed above, our goal is to bring you to optimum levels that can decrease your risk of obesity, diabetes, heart disease, and cancer. It is important to take your Vitamin D with a meal. It is a fat-soluble vitamin that requires fat for the best absorption.

A recent article showed that the combination of low free testosterone and low Vitamin D can be a predictor of mortality in older men. Their conclusion was that a combined deficiency of free testosterone and D3 is significantly associated with heart attacks in a large number of these men. [xxxv]

Question

I've seen the commercials on TV for over-the-counter supplements that claim to increase hormone levels ... and they are a lot cheaper. Are they effective?

There are various over-the-counter pills and treatments that claim to improve men's testosterone levels. And they do ... to an extent. What you need to understand is there are several kinds of testosterone in your body.

You will often hear the term **total testosterone** levels. Testosterone is found in two forms – *free testosterone* and *bound testosterone*. Bound testosterone can be bound to two types of proteins: **albumin** and **sex hormone-binding globulin (SHBG).** It binds tightly to the hormones testosterone, DHT, and estradiol. These proteins transport testosterone throughout the body. About 98% of testosterone is bound to one of these proteins.

The other 2% is known as **free testosterone** and **loosely bound albumin**. This total makes up only 2% of bio-available testosterone. And this is the part that over-the-counter supplements might help restore. But even if it does … it's only 2%.

The important thing to understand here is that all the workouts you do and all the over-the-counter supplements you take will not make your body increase testosterone production in significant levels … because it's only dealing with 2% of the total level. You still wind up with a low overall T score.

Another part of the problem with "just taking some pills" is that you don't know where you started and you don't know where you are. You lack real data. At *The Youth Institute,* we monitor your testosterone levels – from where you start at the very beginning, to where you stay throughout the treatment. That doesn't happen when you buy an over-the-counter supplement.

BHRT does not make your body increase T production. It supplements it. It brings levels back to where they should be … and it keeps them there. That's real health change. That's a difference you will experience. That's getting your body back to the basics.

> *Real health change…. Back to the basics.*

Chapter 5 – How Do I Ge Started?

I trust that I have answered all of your questions by now. If I haven't, please call our office and schedule a consultation. I'll answer any and all questions you have.

Are you ready to begin?

Question

How do I get started? What's the process to go through to become a patient at The Youth Institute?

The Initial Consult

Call our office and set up a consultation appointment. We'll sit down and talk one-on-one in the privacy of my office. Unlike my OB/GYN practice where I have to maintain a strict schedule, I will take as much time as you need to address your concerns.

Sally recently came into my office. She had a lot of questions ... I mean A LOT of questions. She had talked with her personal physician, she had read articles, and she had talked with friends. All that added up to about forty questions she had written down on a legal pad.

We went through them one by one. Several times I pointed her to additional articles that are available on our web site. By the end of our time, I had answered all of her questions. But she still needed some time to decide if BHRT was right for her. I understand those concerns. It's your body. It's your decision. No one can make that decision for you.

Sally called back two days later. We scheduled her for labs, and two days after that she was back in our office receiving pellet placement.

If you talked with her today, she would say, *"That was the best decision I ever made."* But it was made after careful investigation and reflection.

Labs

Let's talk about labs for a minute. The lab tests are very easy and quick. It's a simple blood draw. At this time, we do not do the labs in our offices – there is a lab clinic two minutes away that we recommend. You are usually in-and-out in five to ten minutes. And I receive the results back within 12-24 hours.

Placement

Once I receive your labs, I take those results and personalize a BHRT pellet treatment specifically for you. When you come back in to our office, it takes no more than ten to fifteen minutes for the placement procedure, and then you are good to go.

At that time, our office staff will give you specific instructions for caring for the bandage and tape that protect the incision area.

Follow Through

Our office staff will call you the next day to make sure you are doing well and to answer any other questions you may have at that time.

<table>
<tr><td>Question</td></tr>
</table>

Tell me more about The Youth Institute.
When did you start? What's your history?

The Youth Institute began in Cary, North Carolina five years ago. To date, we have treated over three thousand patients – both men and women. I have patients as young as 18 and, at this point, the oldest is 86.

John's Story

For some people, it takes a while to take that next step. I understand. John Pettit was like that. Here's his story.

"I have talked to Dr. Brannon for too many years about hormone therapy. Honestly, I think the reason I didn't jump in to BHRT was ego. I work in construction; I've always been a "man's man," and I didn't think I needed testosterone. Whatever issues I had physically, I thought I could overcome them on my own. I think there are probably a lot of guys out there who can identify with that attitude.

"Recently, I was at a Christmas party surrounded by many who were patients of Dr. Brannon and were receiving hormone therapy. They all looked fit and trim. They had all lost weight and were in tremendous shape, and to the person, they all talked so positively about it. One of those was a friend of mine who also works in construction. He's definitely a "man's man" who I really respect. He's been on the hormone treatment for three years and told me, "Dude, you just gotta do it!" And I knew it was time.

"I was convinced! I had the pellets done the next week. I know many people do not see changes in their lives as immediately as I did ... but within a week, I could sense a difference. It seemed like my body was being turned into a machine that was much more in sync with itself.

"I am 57 years old and have suffered with ADD for as long as I can remember. The first real change I noticed was that the fog seemed to be lifted in my head. My job in construction

The fog is lifted!

requires me to do some bid work, and a bunch of take-offs (material figuring). Because I've started thinking more clearly, I can set up processes much quicker than before. Now I am usually two or three steps ahead in my mind. The hormone therapy has helped me with my con-centration ten-fold in those areas.

"It has also helped my stamina on the job site. The older I've gotten, the worse my sleep became. I would wake up in the middle of the night and not be able to get back to sleep. No more. With The Youth Institute treatment, I am now sleeping through the night again and waking up refreshed. No more dog-tired, low-energy days.

"I've also had the energy to fly through work outs and am seeing changes in my body shape and muscle tone.

"I know there are a lot of people out there – especially guys – who are hesitant to start. All I can tell you is it's been a game-changer for me. My only regret is that I waited too long to start. My challenge to guys I talk with is to give it a shot. When you look at all you have to gain, I say "Go for it!""

A Final Note

I began this book with you in mind ... engaging in a conversation in my office. This book has answered your questions. I've shown you how you can get your life back through Bio-identical Hormone therapy. The next step is up to you!

I look forward to meeting you personally and helping you get your life back ... to get back to the basics ... to help the new you become the old you (and maybe even better!) ... and to become the healthiest you that you can be.

Give us a call. And check out our web site:

www.TheYouthInstitute.com.

Appendix – Suggested Bibliography

Check It Out for Yourself

Throughout this book, I have encouraged you to do your own research. Don't simply believe what your family physician tells you. Don't believe what you hear on TV or advertisements. And don't even believe me, simply because I've said it.

Truth is truth … and I want you to know the truth … and live by it.

In this appendix, I point you to five key books that show bio-identical hormone replacement therapy is (1) safe, (2) proven, and (3) effective. Check them out!

These books also make reference to hundreds of articles, white papers and research studies that have been done over the years. Look these articles up for yourself. For your convenience, these articles are all also listed on our website, which is continually updated and expanded. You will be able to find them at www.TheYouthInstitute.com where they will be updated continually.

Testosterone for Life: Recharge Your Vitality, Sex Drive, Muscle Mass and Overall Health! Abraham Morgentaler, M.D.

Hormone Optimization in Preventive/Regenerative Medicine, Ron Rothenberg, M.D.

The Youth Effect: A Hormone Therapy Revolution, Ronald L. Brown, M.D.

Greg Brannon, M.D. and *The Youth Institute*

Feel Younger, Stronger, Sexier: The Truth About Bio-Identical Hormones, Dan Hale, M.D.

You Don't Have to Live With It! Uncovering Nature's Power with SottoPelle Bio-Identical Hormones, Gino Tutera, M.D., F.A.C.O.G.

End Notes

[i] Arthur Schopenhauer, as quoted in *The Philosophical Basis of the Conflict Between Liberty and Statism,* Donald w. Miller, Jr., M.D.

[ii] Fournier A, Berrino F, Riboli E, Avenel V, Clavel-Chapelon F. Breast cancer risk in relation to different types of hormone replacement therapy in the E3N-EPIC cohort. Int J Cancer. 2005; 114:448–454.

[iii] Tang M-X, Jacobs D, Stern Y, Marder K, Schofield P, Gurland B 1996 Effect of estrogen during menopause on risk and age at onset of Alzheimer's disease. Lancet 348:429–432.

[iv] Gouras, GK et al. Proc Natl Acad Sci USA, 2000 Feb 1; 97(3):1202-5; Tan, RS, A pilot study on the effects of testosterone in hypogonadal aging male patients with Alzheimer's disease. Aging Male. 2003 Mar; 6(1):13-7.

[v] All of the stories and testimonies that I present in this book are true. At times, I have changed names, dates, and details to protect people's privacy.

[vi] Travison, TB, AB Araujo, AB O'Donnell, V Kupelian, JB McKinlay, 2007. A population-level decline in seum testosterone levels in American men. *Journal of Clinical Endocrinology and Metabolism 92:196-202.*

[vii] Dirty Dozen Endocrine Disruptors: 12 Hormone-Altering Chemicals and How to Avoid Them, http://www.ewg.org/research/dirty-dozen-list-endocrine-disruptors?gclid=CjwKEAiA3NTFBRDKheuO6IG43VQSJAA74F77I2uDCgoZKK5FNBvvrkJVF3-NmbOrfcCj7_LMG5o-yBoC9ZDw_wcB

[viii] Ibid.

[ix] Kathleen Doheny, Statins May Lower Testosterone, Libido, WebMD, http://www.webmd.com/erectile-dysfunction/news/20100416/statins_may_lower_testosterone_libido; Sayer Ji, Do Cholesterol Drugs Have Men by their Gonads? GreenMedInfo, LLC., http://www.greenmedinfo.com/blog/do-cholesterol-drugs-have-men-their-gonads; Schooling CM, et al. BMC Med. 2013, The effect of statins on testosterone in men and women, a systematic review and meta-analysis of randomized controlled trials, PubMed, https://www.ncbi.nlm.nih.gov/m/pubmed/23448151.

[x] Khaw KT, Dowsett M, Folkerd E, et al. Endogenous testosterone and mortality due to all causes, cardiovascular disease, and cancer in men: European prospective investigation into cancer in Norfolk (EPIC-Norfolk) Prospective Population Study. Circulation. 2007;116(23):2694–2701.

[xi] Korenman SG, Morley JE, Mooradian AD, et al. 1990 Secondary hypogonadism in older men: its relationship to impotence. 3 Clin Endocrinol Metab. 71:963-969.

[xii] Shores MM, Matsumoto AM, Sloan KL, Kivlahan DR. Low serum testosterone and mortality in male veterans. Arch Intern Med. 2006;166(15):1660–1665.

[xiii] Hak AE, Witteman JC, de Jong FH, et al. Low levels of endogenous androgens increase the risk of atherosclerosis in elderly men: the Rotterdam study. J Clin Endocrinol Metab2002; 87:3632–9.)

[xiv] Testosterone for Life Abraham Morgentaler, MD McGraw Hill copyright 2009 page 53.

[xv] Men with coronary artery disease have lower levels of androgens than men with normal coronary angiograms K. M. English, O. Mandour, R. P. Steeds, M. J. Diver, T. H. Jones and K. S. Channer Department of Clinical Chemistry, Royal Liverpool University Hospital, Liverpool, U.K.

[xvi] Testosterone Therapy in Women with Chronic Heart Failure: A Pilot Double-blind, Randomized, Placebo-controlled Study Ferdinando Iellamo, MD, Maurizio Volterrani, MD, Giuseppe Caminiti, MD, Roger Karam, MD, Rosalba Massaro, MD, Massimo Fini, MD, Peter Collins, MD, PhD, Giuseppe M.C. Rosano, MD J Am Coll Cardiol. 2010;56(16):1310-1316. Journal of the American College of Cardiology.

[xvii] Testosterone replacement in hypogonadal men with angina improves ischemic threshold and quality of life Heart 2004; 90:871-876 doi:10.1136/hrt.2003.021121 Cardiovascular medicine C J Malkin, P J Pugh, P D Morris, K E Kerry, R D Jones, T H Jones,K S Channer.

[xviii] Mayo Clinic Proceedings, January 2000.

[xix] The Journal of the National Cancer Institute, 2008.

[xx] Morgentaler, ibid, page 116-128.

[xxi] Morgentaler, ibid, page 125.

[xxii] Johnell O and Kanis JA (2006) An estimate of the worldwide prevalence and disability associated with osteoporotic fractures. Osteoporos Int 17:1726.

[xxiii] Kanis JA (2007) WHO Technical Report, University of Sheffield, UK: 66.

[xxiv] EFFO and NOF (1997) Who are candidates for prevention and treatment for osteoporosis? Osteoporos Int 7:1.

[xxv] Johnell O and Kanis JA (2006) An estimate of the worldwide prevalence and disability associated with osteoporotic fractures. Osteoporos Int 17:1726.

[xxvi] Melton LJ, 3rd, Atkinson EJ, O'Connor MK, et al. (1998) Bone density and fracture risk in men. J Bone Miner Res 13:1915; Melton LJ, 3rd, Chrischilles EA, Cooper C, et al. (1992) Perspective. How many women have osteoporosis? J Bone Miner Res 7:1005; Kanis JA, Johnell O, Oden A, et al. (2000) Long-term risk of osteoporotic fracture in Malmo. Osteoporos Int 11:669.

[xxvii] Studd, J WW, et al (1990) Am Journal OB/GYN 163, 1474-1479; Christiansen et al, 1981; Lindsay et al, 1976; Stevenson et al, 1990.

[xxviii] Fournier A, Berrino F, Riboli E, Avenel V, Clavel-Chapelon F. Breast cancer risk in relation to different types of hormone replacement therapy in the E3N-EPIC cohort. Int J Cancer. 2005; 114:448–454.

[xxix] Bioidentical Hormone Therapy Mayo Clinic Procedure July 2011.

[xxx] The Hormone Solution, Stay Younger Longer with Natural Hormone and Nutrition Therapies Thierry Hertoghe, MD Copyright 2002 Three Rivers Press.

[xxxi] Fournier A, ibid. pages 114:448–454.

[xxxii] Morgentaler, ibid.

[xxxiii] Khaw, ibid.

[xxxiv] The following information is taken from an article by *The Youth Institute* entited *Vitamin D3*.

[xxxv] Lerchbaum E, et al. Clin Endocrinol (Oxf). 2012 Sep;77(3):475-83. doi: 10.1111/j.1365-2265.2012.04371.x.

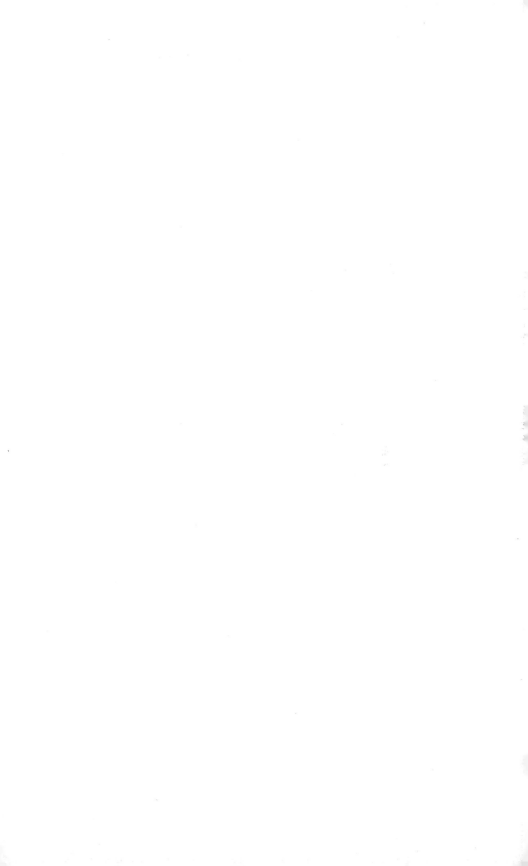

Made in the USA
Columbia, SC
04 June 2018